LIVING AND THRIVING WITH DIABETES

DR DECLAN HARVEY

Table of Contents

CHAPTER ONE

INTRODUCTION

Diabetes is a metabolic disorder characterized by high levels of glucose in the blood. It occurs when the body is unable to properly produce or use insulin, a hormone that regulates blood sugar levels.

There are two types of diabetes: type 1 and type 2. Type 1 diabetes is an autoimmune disease in which the body's immune system attacks and destroys the cells in the pancreas that produce insulin. This results in little to no insulin production, leading to high blood sugar levels. Type 2 diabetes, on the other hand, occurs when the body becomes insulin resistant, meaning it does not respond properly to insulin. This causes high blood sugar levels as well.

The main physiological changes that occur with diabetes include:

- Insufficient insulin production or response: In

type 1 diabetes, the body's immune system destroys the insulin-producing cells in the pancreas, leading to little to no insulin production. In type 2 diabetes, the body becomes resistant to the effects of insulin, causing it to produce less insulin or not use it efficiently.

- Elevated blood sugar levels: Insulin is responsible for transporting glucose from the blood into cells for energy. With insufficient insulin, glucose accumulates in the blood, leading to high blood sugar levels.

- Imbalance in energy production: When there is not enough insulin to transport glucose into cells, the body cannot use it for energy. As a result, the body turns to alternative sources of energy, such as breaking down fat and protein. This can lead to weight loss and muscle wasting.
- Dehydration and increased thirst: High levels of blood

sugar can cause the body to try to flush out the excess sugar through urination, leading to dehydration. This can also cause increased thirst as the body tries to replenish lost fluids.

- Increased hunger: With insufficient insulin, the body cannot properly use glucose for energy. As a result, it may trigger hunger signals, leading to increased appetite and weight gain.

- Fatigue: Without enough glucose reaching the cells for energy production, the body may experience fatigue and weakness.
- Damage to blood vessels and nerves: Over time, high blood sugar levels can damage the blood vessels and nerves, leading to various complications, such as heart disease, kidney disease, nerve damage, and vision problems.
- Increased risk of infection: High blood sugar levels can weaken the immune

system, making individuals with diabetes more susceptible to infections and slower to heal from injuries.

UNDERSTANDING DIABETES

Importance of Understanding Diabetes

- Manage the Condition effectively: Understanding diabetes is crucial for managing the condition effectively. With proper knowledge, individuals with diabetes can learn how to monitor their blood sugar levels, take their medication, exercise, and make dietary changes to keep their diabetes under control.

- Prevent Complications: Diabetes is a chronic condition that can lead to serious complications such as heart disease, stroke, nerve damage, and kidney disease. By understanding diabetes, individuals can take steps to prevent or delay these complications and improve their overall health.

- Make Informed Decisions: Knowing the facts about diabetes allows individuals to make informed decisions about their health. This includes understanding the risks associated with the condition, knowing how to prevent or manage it, and being aware of the available treatment options.
- Recognize Symptoms: Knowing the symptoms of

diabetes is crucial for early detection and treatment. Understanding how diabetes affects the body can help individuals recognize and report any symptoms they may experience, leading to earlier diagnosis and better management of the condition.

- Support System: Understanding diabetes can also help family and friends provide better support to their loved ones with diabetes. By learning about the condition, they can offer emotional support and help with managing the daily challenges of living with diabetes.

- Better Quality of Life: With proper management, individuals with diabetes can live a normal and healthy life. Understanding the condition can help them make the necessary lifestyle changes to improve their overall health and quality of life.
- Lower Healthcare Costs: By understanding diabetes and

effectively managing it, individuals can potentially lower their healthcare costs. This is because they are less likely to develop complications that require hospitalization or other expensive treatments.

Causes of diabetes

- Genetics: Certain genetic factors can increase a person's risk of developing diabetes. Having a family history of diabetes, especially in a first-degree relative, can increase the likelihood of developing the disease.

- Obesity and sedentary lifestyle: Being overweight or obese can increase the risk of developing type 2 diabetes. This is because excess weight can make it more difficult for the body to use insulin effectively, leading to insulin resistance. Similarly, a sedentary lifestyle, with little or no physical activity, can also contribute to insulin resistance and the development of type 2 diabetes.

- Insulin resistance: In type 2 diabetes, the body's cells become resistant to insulin, meaning they are unable to use it effectively. This leads to high blood sugar levels, as the body is not able to properly regulate glucose.

- Autoimmune response: In type 1 diabetes, the body's immune system attacks and destroys the cells in the pancreas that produce insulin. This results in the body's inability to produce insulin, leading to high blood sugar levels.

- Pancreatic damage or disease: In some cases, damage to the pancreas due to injury, infection, or certain diseases can lead to the development of diabetes.

SYMPTOMS OF DIABETES

- Frequent urination: One of the main symptoms of diabetes is frequent urination. This is because high blood sugar levels can interfere with the kidneys' ability to properly reabsorb fluids.

- Extreme thirst: Due to frequent urination, people with diabetes may experience extreme thirst and may feel the need to drink large amounts of water.

- Increased hunger: As the body struggles to regulate its blood sugar levels, people with diabetes may experience increased hunger and may feel the need to eat more often.

- Unexplained weight loss: Despite an increased appetite, some people with diabetes may experience sudden and unexplained weight loss. This is because the body is not able to properly utilize glucose for energy and starts breaking down fat and muscle for fuel.
- Fatigue: In addition to weight loss, high blood sugar levels can also cause feelings of fatigue and weakness.

- Numbness and tingling in hands and feet: High blood sugar levels can cause nerve damage in the body, leading to numbness and tingling in the extremities, particularly in the hands and feet.

CHAPTER TWO

MANAGING DIABETES

There are different ways by which one can manage diabetes and it includes:

1) HEALTHY EATING HABITS

- Plan your meals: Create a meal plan that includes a variety of healthy foods from all food groups. This will ensure that you are getting a balanced and nutritious diet.

- Choose healthy carbohydrates: Carbohydrates can raise blood sugar levels, so it's important to choose healthy ones like whole grains, fruits, vegetables, and legumes.
- Control portion sizes: Overeating can lead to high blood sugar levels, so it's important to control your portion sizes and aim for smaller, more frequent meals.
- Monitor your sugar intake: Limit your consumption of

added sugars and sugary drinks. Instead, choose natural sweeteners like fruits or use low-calorie sweeteners in moderation.

- Eat lots of fruits and vegetables: These are packed with vitamins, minerals, and fiber, which can help control blood sugar levels and improve overall health.
- Choose lean proteins: Lean proteins like poultry, fish, and plant-based sources like tofu and beans are

lower in fat and can help manage blood sugar levels.

- Choose healthy fats: Healthy fats like avocados, nuts, and olive oil can have a positive impact on blood sugar and heart health.
- Limit processed foods: Processed foods are often high in added sugars, unhealthy fats, and sodium, all of which can negatively affect blood sugar levels.

2) Regular exercise

Regular exercise is an essential part of managing

diabetes. It can help control blood sugar levels, improve insulin sensitivity, and reduce the risk of complications related to diabetes. Here are some tips for incorporating regular exercise into your diabetes management plan:

- Consult with your doctor: Before starting any exercise program, it is important to consult with your doctor. They can assess your overall health and provide personalized recommendations for the

type and intensity of exercise that is suitable for you.

- Choose activities you enjoy: Find activities that you enjoy doing, such as walking, swimming, biking, or dancing. This will make it easier to stick to a regular exercise routine and prevent boredom.

- Set realistic goals: Start with small, achievable goals and gradually work your way up to more challenging ones. This will help you stay motivated and prevent burnout or injury.

- Monitor your blood sugar levels: It is important to check your blood sugar levels before, during, and after exercise, especially if you are taking insulin or other medications that can lower your blood sugar. If your blood sugar levels are too high or too low, adjust your exercise intensity or have a light snack to bring them back to normal.
- Stay hydrated: Drink plenty of water before, during,

and after exercise to prevent dehydration. Dehydration can cause blood sugar levels to rise, so it is important to stay hydrated while exercising.

- Have a snack before and after exercise: Eating a healthy snack before and after exercise can help prevent low blood sugar levels and provide energy for your workout. Choose a snack that is high in protein and complex carbohydrates, such as a piece of fruit with a handful of nuts.

- Be prepared for emergencies: Always carry a source of fast-acting carbohydrates with you while exercising, such as a glucose tablet or juice, in case of a low blood sugar emergency.
- Listen to your body: If you experience any symptoms of low blood sugar, such as dizziness, shakiness, or confusion, stop exercising and treat the low blood sugar immediately. If you

are feeling unwell or have any other symptoms, stop exercising and consult with your doctor.

- Don't forget strength training: Incorporate strength training exercises into your routine to help build muscle and improve insulin sensitivity. This can be done using weights, resistance bands, or bodyweight exercises.
- Stay consistent: Consistency is key when it comes to managing diabetes with exercise. Aim

for at least 30 minutes of moderate-intensity exercise, such as brisk walking, five days a week.

3) By monitoring blood sugar

- Regularly check blood sugar levels: Use a glucometer to test blood sugar levels at least 2-4 times a day, or as recommended by a healthcare provider. Record the results in a logbook to track patterns and identify any potential issues.

- Know your target range:
  Work with a healthcare
  provider to determine your
  target blood sugar range.
  This will vary depending on
  individual factors such as
  age, lifestyle, and overall
  health.
- Adjust diet: Follow a
  balanced, healthy diet that
  is low in sugar and
  carbohydrates. Limit or
  avoid foods that can cause
  a spike in blood sugar
  levels. Consider consulting
  with a registered dietitian

for personalized meal planning.

- Take medication as prescribed: If prescribed insulin or other diabetes medications, take them as directed by a healthcare provider. Monitor blood sugar levels regularly, and if levels are consistently outside of the target range, talk to a healthcare provider about adjusting medication dosage.
- Exercise regularly: Physical activity can help lower blood sugar levels and

improve overall health. Aim for at least 30 minutes of moderate exercise, such as brisk walking, most days of the week.

- Stay hydrated: Drink plenty of water throughout the day to stay hydrated and help regulate blood sugar levels.
- Keep stress levels under control: Stress can affect blood sugar levels in some individuals. Consider practicing stress-reducing techniques, such as deep

breathing, yoga, or meditation.

- Regular check-ups: Schedule regular check-ups with a healthcare provider to monitor overall health and diabetes management. They can also provide guidance on adjusting treatment plans if needed.
- Monitor for symptoms: Pay attention to any changes in symptoms, such as frequent urination, excessive thirst, hunger, fatigue, or blurred vision. These could be signs of

high or low blood sugar levels and may require immediate attention.

- Educate yourself: Stay informed about the latest research and recommendations for managing diabetes. Attend diabetes education classes, join support groups, and talk to healthcare providers about any questions or concerns you may have.

4) Medications and insulin

Diabetes is a chronic condition that affects how the body

processes glucose, or sugar, in the blood. In order to effectively manage diabetes, it is important to closely monitor blood sugar levels and maintain them within a healthy range. This can be achieved through the use of medication and/or insulin.

Medication is often used in the management of diabetes to help the body better regulate blood sugar levels. There are different types of medication that may be prescribed, depending on the type of diabetes a person has and their individual needs. Some common types of diabetes medication include:

1. Metformin: This medication works by decreasing the amount of glucose produced by the liver and increasing the body's sensitivity to insulin.

2. Sulfonylureas: These medications stimulate the pancreas to produce more insulin, helping to lower blood sugar levels.

3. Thiazolidinediones: These medications also work to increase the body's sensitivity to insulin, helping to control blood sugar levels.

4. DPP-4 inhibitors: These drugs help to lower blood sugar levels by preventing the breakdown of certain hormones that increase insulin production.

5. GLP-1 receptor agonists: These injectable drugs work by slowing down digestion, which in turn helps to control blood sugar levels.

6. SGLT2 inhibitors: These medications help the kidneys to remove excess sugar from the blood, which can lower blood sugar levels.

In some cases, medication alone may not be enough to adequately control blood sugar levels. In these cases, insulin therapy may also be necessary. Insulin is a hormone that is normally produced by the pancreas, and it helps to regulate blood sugar levels. People with type 1 diabetes do not produce enough insulin and therefore require insulin therapy. Some people with type 2 diabetes may also need to use insulin in addition to medication or if their diabetes becomes more difficult to manage.

Insulin therapy involves injecting insulin into the body using a syringe, insulin pen, or insulin pump. The type of insulin and the frequency of injections will depend on an individual's specific needs and diabetes management plan.

Managing diabetes through medication and insulin also involves regularly checking blood sugar levels, following a healthy diet, and staying physically active. It is important to work closely with a healthcare team to determine the best treatment plan and to make any necessary adjustments over time. With proper management, people with diabetes can lead healthy and fulfilling lives.

TIPS FOR DAILY LIVING WITH DIABETES

Although a few of the tips that would be listed below has been aforementioned under different subtopics, we would be reiterating on a few of them as they are important for daily living with diabetes.

- Keep track of your blood sugar levels: Monitoring your blood sugar levels regularly can help you understand how your body responds to different foods, activities, and medication. This can help you make necessary adjustments to your daily routine to keep your levels stable.

- Follow a healthy diet: A nutritious and balanced diet is crucial for managing diabetes. Choose foods that are low in sugar, saturated fats, and processed carbohydrates. Focus on incorporating more fruits, vegetables, whole grains, and lean proteins into your meals.

- Stay physically active: Regular exercise can help improve insulin sensitivity and manage blood sugar levels. Aim for at least 30 minutes of moderate exercise every day, such as brisk walking, cycling, or swimming.

- Monitor your medication intake: If you take medication for diabetes, make sure to take it as prescribed by your doctor. It's also essential to keep track of any side effects or changes in your blood sugar levels to discuss with your healthcare team.

- Prioritize stress management: High levels of stress can cause blood sugar levels to rise. Find healthy ways to manage stress, such as yoga, meditation, or talking to a trusted friend or therapist.
- Don't skip meals: Skipping meals, especially breakfast, can lead to blood sugar fluctuations. Stick to a regular eating schedule, and make sure to have

healthy snacks on hand if needed.

- Stay hydrated: Drinking enough water is essential for overall health and managing diabetes. Aim for at least 8 glasses of water per day and limit sugary drinks.

- Get enough sleep: Lack of sleep can affect your blood sugar levels and make it harder to manage diabetes. Aim for 7-9 hours of quality sleep each night.

- Educate yourself: Stay informed about your

diabetes and how to manage it. Attend educational classes, seminars, or workshops on the latest research and tips for living with diabetes.

- Don't be afraid to ask for help: Managing diabetes can be challenging, and it's okay to ask for help when needed. Lean on your support system, whether it's family, friends, or your healthcare team, for encouragement and guidance.

CHAPTER THREE

LIVING A FULL LIFE WITH DIABETES

The fact that you have diabetes doesn't mean you are no longer a normal human as you can still go about your life activities like every other person. Here, we would discuss a few life activities that diabetic patients can take part in while taking precautions.

1) Travelling with diabetes

- Consult with your doctor: Before embarking on your trip, make sure to consult with your doctor to discuss any concerns or specific instructions for managing your diabetes while traveling. Your doctor can also provide a letter outlining your condition and any necessary medications or supplies you may need.
- Pack extra medication and supplies: It's important to pack more than enough of your diabetes medications, including insulin, test

strips, and glucose monitoring devices. This is in case of unexpected delays or loss of medication during your trip.

- Keep medication and supplies with you: It is recommended to keep your medication and diabetes supplies with you in your carry-on luggage rather than in your checked baggage. This way, you have immediate access to them in case of any emergencies or delays.

- Make sure to monitor your blood sugar regularly: Traveling can disrupt your usual routine, which can affect your blood sugar levels. Make sure to check your blood sugar frequently and adjust your medication and insulin dosages accordingly.

- Stay hydrated and avoid sugary drinks: It's important to stay hydrated while traveling, especially if you're flying. Opt for water instead of sugary drinks to avoid spikes in your blood sugar levels.

- Be mindful of meal options: If you have specific dietary restrictions due to your diabetes, research the meal options available at your travel destination. This will help you plan ahead and avoid any difficulties in finding suitable meals.

- Wear a medical alert bracelet: In case of any emergencies, it's important to wear a medical alert bracelet that identifies you as a person with diabetes.

This will help first responders provide appropriate care in case you're unable to communicate.

- Plan for potential insulin storage: If you're traveling to a location with extreme temperatures, you may need to find a way to keep your insulin at the recommended storage temperature. This could mean packing a cool pack or finding a refrigerator at your accommodation.

- Prepare for time zone changes: If you're traveling to a different time zone, discuss with your doctor how to adjust your medication schedule accordingly. You may also need to monitor your blood sugar levels more frequently during the first few days of your trip.

2) Maintaining social relationships

Living with diabetes brings about a unique set of challenges, and maintaining a social relationship can be one of them. It requires managing your blood sugar levels while also navigating social events and interactions. However, it is important to remember that living with diabetes does not mean you have to sacrifice your social life. Here are some tips for managing diabetes while maintaining a fulfilling social life.

- Educate your friends and loved ones about diabetes : One of the first steps in maintaining a social relationship while living with diabetes is to educate your friends and loved ones about your condition. Let them know what diabetes is, how it affects you, and what they can do to support you. This will not only help them understand your needs better but also make them more mindful of how their actions may impact your health.

- Plan ahead : It's essential to plan ahead when it comes to managing your diabetes in social situations. If you know you'll be attending an event with food, make a plan on what and how much you will eat. If necessary, bring your own snacks or ask the host about the menu beforehand. Planning ahead can help you stay in control of your blood sugar levels while still enjoying social gatherings.

- Communicate with your friends and loved ones : Communication is key in any relationship, and it becomes even more important when managing diabetes. It's essential to communicate with your friends and loved ones about your needs, such as taking breaks to check your blood sugar or stepping away to administer insulin. Let them know that their support is essential to managing your condition, and they will likely be happy to accommodate your needs.

- Don't be afraid to say no: While it's crucial to maintain a social life, it's also important to prioritize your health. If you feel overwhelmed or unwell, don't be afraid to say no to social events or activities. Your friends and loved ones will understand and support your decision to take care of yourself.

- Make healthy choices: Social situations can often involve unhealthy food and drinks, which can be challenging to resist. However, it's essential to make healthy choices for managing your diabetes.

Opt for healthier options like salads, grilled chicken, and water instead of sugary drinks or fried foods. Be mindful of your portion sizes and try to eat at regular intervals to keep your blood sugar levels stable.

- Be prepared for emergencies: Sometimes, despite our best efforts, unexpected situations can arise. It's important to be prepared for emergencies by carrying essentials such as glucose tablets, insulin, and a blood glucose monitor with you at all times. Let your friends and loved ones know where you keep these items in case of an emergency.

Living with diabetes can be challenging, but it should not stop you from maintaining a social relationship. By educating yourself and the people around you, planning ahead, and making healthy choices, you can successfully manage your diabetes while still enjoying a fulfilling social life. Remember to prioritize your health and communicate your needs, and your friends and loved ones will support and understand your condition.

3) Taking care of other health conditions

Living with diabetes can be a daily challenge, but when you also have other health conditions to manage, it can often feel overwhelming. Balancing the needs and demands of multiple health conditions can be a difficult task, but with some careful planning and self-care, it is possible to live a fulfilling life while keeping all your conditions under control.

First and foremost, communication with your healthcare team is crucial. It is important to keep them informed about all of your health conditions and any related medications you may be taking. This will help them to create a comprehensive treatment plan that takes into account all of your conditions and helps you manage them effectively.

One of the biggest challenges of living with multiple health conditions is managing different dietary restrictions and medications. In the case of diabetes, it is essential to maintain a healthy diet and monitor blood sugar levels closely. However, if you have other conditions such as high blood pressure or kidney disease, you may also need to follow specific dietary restrictions. It is important to work with your healthcare team or a registered dietitian to create a meal plan that meets all of your nutritional needs.

Taking medication can also become more complicated when you have multiple health conditions. It is important to keep a list of all your medications, including the dosages, schedules, and potential side effects. This will help you and your healthcare team monitor for any potential interactions between your medications and make adjustments as needed. It is also essential to never skip or stop taking medication without consulting your doctor, as it can have serious consequences for your health.

In addition to managing your physical health, it is also crucial to prioritize your mental health. Living with multiple health conditions can be emotionally draining, and it is important to take breaks and engage in activities that bring you joy and reduce stress. This could be anything from reading a book, spending time with loved ones, or practicing relaxation techniques such as yoga or deep breathing. Taking care of your mental health is just as important as taking care of your physical health and can also have a positive impact on your overall well-being.

Furthermore, attending regular check-ups and screenings is vital for managing your health conditions. Your healthcare team may recommend that you visit different specialists for each of your conditions, so it is crucial to keep track of all appointments and keep open communication between them. This will ensure that all aspects of your health are being monitored and addressed.

Finally, it is essential to remember that living with multiple health conditions does not define you. It is important to focus on the things you can control, such as following your treatment plan and making healthy lifestyle choices. Reach out to support groups or friends who understand your struggles and can offer support and encouragement. Remember to celebrate your successes, even if they seem small, and practice self-care regularly.

Living with diabetes while managing other health conditions can be challenging, but it is possible to find a balance and live a fulfilling life. With open communication, careful planning, and self-care, you can effectively manage all of your health conditions and maintain your overall well-being. Remember to prioritize your health, both physical and mental, and never be afraid to ask for help when needed. You are not alone in your journey, and with the right support, you can thrive despite any challenges that may arise.

CHAPTER FOUR

CONCLUSION

Thriving with diabetes

Living with diabetes can be challenging, but it does not mean that one cannot lead a fulfilling and thriving life. With proper management and a positive mindset, individuals with diabetes can thrive in all aspects of life.

One of the key factors in thriving with diabetes is education and understanding.

It is important to learn about the disease, its management, and potential complications. This knowledge empowers individuals to take control of their health and make informed decisions. It also helps in developing a personalized management plan in consultation with healthcare professionals.

Another crucial aspect is self-care. It is essential to prioritize self-care, including maintaining a healthy diet, regular physical activity, and proper medication adherence. Taking care of one's mental and emotional health is also crucial. Stress management techniques, such as meditation, deep breathing, and talking to a therapist, can be helpful in coping with the challenges of living with diabetes.

One of the biggest challenges for individuals with diabetes is managing blood sugar levels. It is essential to consistently monitor blood sugar levels and adjust medications accordingly. Keeping a record of blood sugar levels can also help identify patterns and make necessary changes to the management plan.

It is also important to have a support system in place. Family, friends, and support groups can provide emotional support and practical help in managing diabetes. They can also be a source of motivation and accountability in keeping up with healthy lifestyle habits.

Positive thinking and a can-do attitude can also go a long way in thriving with diabetes. Instead of focusing on the limitations and challenges, it is important to prioritize the things that can be controlled. Set realistic goals and celebrate small victories, whether it is maintaining a healthy blood sugar level or completing a physical activity.

Having diabetes may also require some adjustments in daily life, but it does not mean giving up on things that bring joy and fulfillment. With proper management and planning, individuals with diabetes can still pursue their passions and lead a fulfilling life. It is important to find a balance between managing diabetes and enjoying life to the fullest.

Finally, it is imperative to never underestimate the power of a positive mindset. Instead of viewing diabetes as a barrier, see it as an opportunity to make positive changes in life. With the right mindset, individuals with diabetes can thrive and achieve their full potential in all aspects of life.

In conclusion, having diabetes isn't the end of the world as you have learnt from the book that you are not different from those who are free from it so go and thrive even as you **LIVE WITH DIABETES**

THE END